TYPE 1 DIABETIC VEGETARIAN RECIPES FOR KIDS

Managing Type 1 Diabetes with Plant-Based Recipes Kids Will Love

By Mia Bennett

COPYRIGHT PAGE

All rights reserved. The copyright holder must provide written permission before any part of this publication can be republished in any manner, such as photocopying, scanning, or other methods.

Copyright ©2024

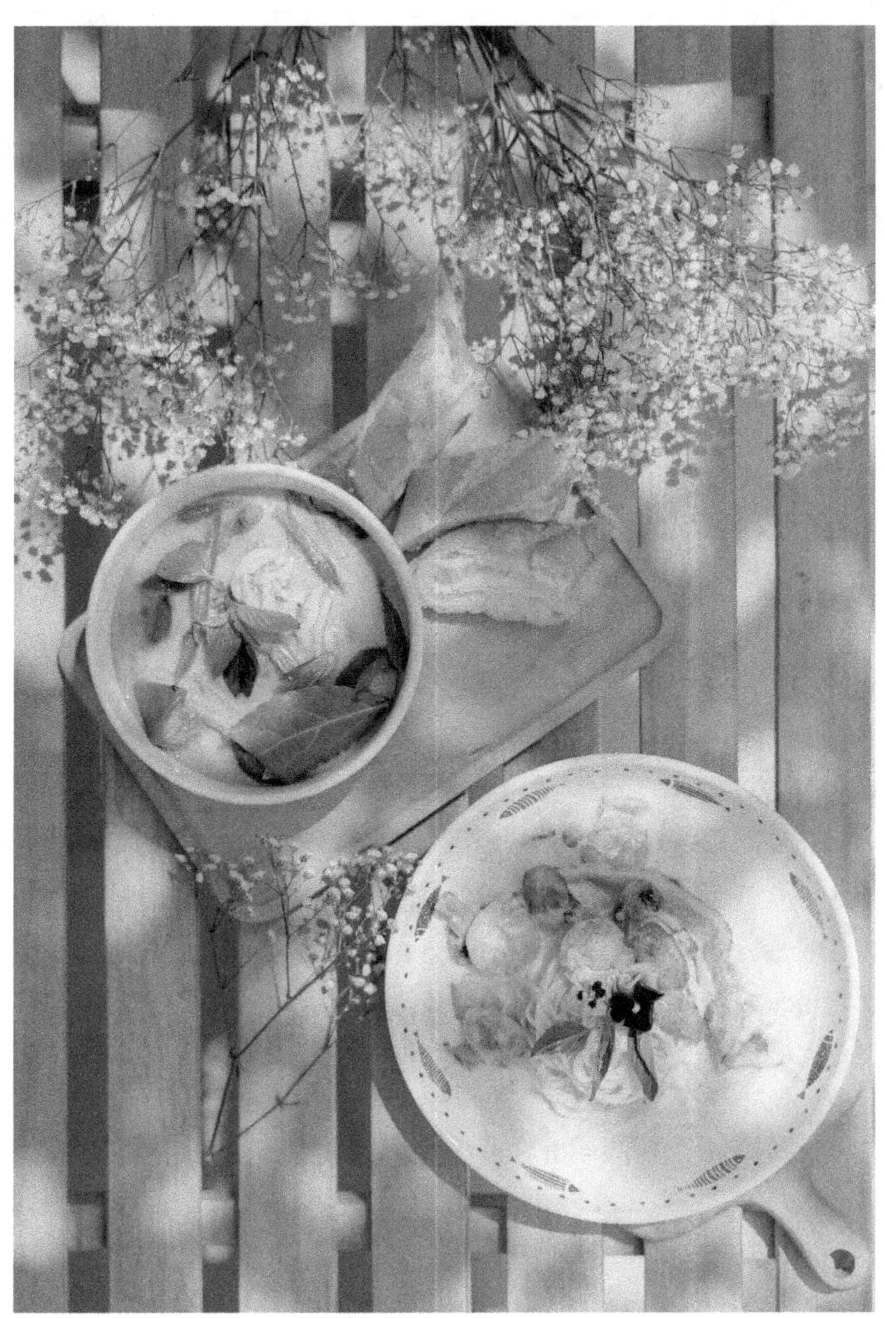

TABLE OF CONTENTS

Chapter 3: Lunch Recipes 38

Chapter 4: Dinner Recipes 57

INTRODUCTION

I magine this: your energetic child, full of life and questions, has just been diagnosed with type 1 diabetes (T1D). It's a whirlwind of emotions, but amidst it all, there's a unique aspect to consider – your family follows a vegetarian diet. Fear not, this guide will equip you with the knowledge to navigate T1D management alongside a plant-based lifestyle for your child.

Understanding Type 1 Diabetes in Children:

Unlike type 2 diabetes, T1D is an autoimmune condition where the body attacks insulin-producing cells in the pancreas. Insulin is a key player, unlocking the door for glucose (sugar) to enter cells and provide energy. Without enough insulin, blood sugar levels rise, leading to a cascade of health problems if left unchecked.

Nutritional Needs of Vegetarian Kids with T1D:

The good news? A well-planned vegetarian diet can be incredibly beneficial for managing T1D. Here's why:

- **Fiber Powerhouse:** Plant-based meals are typically rich in fiber, which helps slow down carbohydrate absorption and prevent blood sugar spikes.
- **Weight Management:** Vegetarian diets tend to be lower in saturated fat, promoting healthy weight management, another crucial factor in T1D control.
- **Nutrient Rich**: Fruits, vegetables, legumes, and whole grains offer a spectrum of vitamins and minerals essential for a growing child.

However, there are some considerations:

- **Protein Power**: Vegetarian diets, especially lacto-ovo (including dairy and eggs), can provide sufficient protein, but plan meals with variety (lentils, tofu, nuts) to ensure all essential amino acids are met.
- **Iron and Vitamin B12**: These nutrients are more readily available in animal products. Consult your pediatrician about incorporating fortified foods or supplements.

Tips for Meal Planning and Preparation:

- **Carb Counting is Key**: Work with a registered dietitian to learn carb counting, a method to estimate carbohydrate content in food and adjust insulin doses accordingly.

- **Focus on Complex Carbs:** Prioritize whole grains, vegetables, and legumes over refined carbohydrates like white bread or sugary drinks. These release glucose slower, minimizing blood sugar spikes.

- **Pair Carbs with Protein and Fat**: Combining carbs with protein and healthy fats (avocado, nuts) promotes satiety and helps regulate blood sugar levels.

- **Snack Savvy:** Plan regular snacks with a balance of carbs, protein, and healthy fats to prevent hypoglycemia (low blood sugar). Think veggie sticks with hummus, whole-wheat crackers with cheese, or a handful of nuts and dried fruit.

- **Get Creative in the Kitchen:** Involve your child in meal planning and preparation. Explore vegetarian recipes online or in cookbooks. Let them choose colorful vegetables, experiment with spices, and create fun food presentations.

- **Embrace Flexibility:** Life throws curveballs – unexpected activities or social gatherings can disrupt meal plans.Pack healthy snacks, have backup options, and adjust insulin as needed.

Remember: You're not alone! By working as a team, you can empower your child to manage their diabetes effectively while embracing a healthy, plant-based lifestyle.

Chapter 1: 30-Day Meal Plan

Week 1:

Day 1

- Breakfast: Veggie Scramble with Tofu
- Lunch: Chickpea and Avocado Salad
- Dinner: Eggplant Parmesan
- Snack: Roasted Chickpeas
- Dessert: Apple Cinnamon Oat Bars

Day 2

- Breakfast: Berry Oatmeal with Chia Seeds
- Lunch: Lentil Soup with Vegetables
- Dinner: Vegetable Stir-Fry with Tofu
- Snack: Veggie Sticks with Hummus
- Dessert: Baked Pears with Cinnamon

Day 3

- Breakfast: Spinach and Mushroom Omelette
- Lunch: Quinoa and Black Bean Salad
- Dinner: Spinach and Ricotta Stuffed Shells
- Snack: Baked Zucchini Chips
- Dessert: Greek Yogurt with Honey and Berries

Day 4

- Breakfast: Whole Grain Pancakes with Almond Butter
- Lunch: Grilled Veggie Wraps
- Dinner: Black Bean and Sweet Potato Enchiladas
- Snack: Edamame with Sea Salt
- Dessert: Vegan Chocolate Avocado Mousse

Day 5

- Breakfast: Greek Yogurt Parfait with Mixed Berries
- Lunch: Spinach and Feta Stuffed Peppers
- Dinner: Veggie Burger with Whole Wheat Bun
- Snack: Apple Slices with Almond Butter
- Dessert: Chia Seed Pudding with Mango

Day 6

- Breakfast: Avocado Toast with Tomato and Basil
- Lunch: Tomato and Basil Soup
- Dinner: Stuffed Bell Peppers with Quinoa
- Snack: Cucumber and Tomato Salad
- Dessert: Mixed Berry Sorbet

Day 7

- Breakfast: Quinoa Breakfast Bowl with Apples and Cinnamon

- Lunch: Veggie Sushi Rolls
- Dinner: Cauliflower Pizza with Veggie Toppings
- Snack: Spinach Artichoke Dip with Whole Grain Crackers
- Dessert: Almond Flour Cookies

Week 2:

Day 8

- Breakfast: Smoothie Bowl with Nuts and Seeds
- Lunch: Greek Salad with Tofu
- Dinner: Ratatouille with Brown Rice
- Snack: Veggie Spring Rolls
- Dessert: Frozen Banana Pops

Day 9

- Breakfast: Sweet Potato Hash with Bell Peppers
- Lunch: Hummus and Veggie Sandwich
- Dinner: Lentil Tacos with Avocado Salsa
- Snack: Sweet Potato Fries
- Dessert: Coconut Macaroons

Day 10

- Breakfast: Cottage Cheese and Fruit Salad
- Lunch: Zucchini Noodles with Pesto

- Dinner: Baked Ziti with Spinach
- Snack: Guacamole with Veggie Dippers
- Dessert: Pumpkin Spice Energy Balls

Day 11

- Breakfast: Vegan Banana Muffins
- Lunch: Stuffed Acorn Squash
- Dinner: Butternut Squash Risotto
- Snack: Mini Caprese Skewers
- Dessert: Lemon Chia Seed Muffins

Day 12

- Breakfast: Whole Wheat Waffles with Fresh Berries
- Lunch: Mushroom and Barley Stew
- Dinner: Broccoli and Cheddar Stuffed Potatoes
- Snack: Carrot and Oat Cookies
- Dessert: Fruit Salad with Mint

Day 13

- Breakfast: Chia Seed Pudding with Coconut Milk
- Lunch: Caprese Salad with Balsamic Glaze
- Dinner: Portobello Mushroom Fajitas
- Snack: Cauliflower Buffalo Wings
- Dessert: Dark Chocolate Dipped Strawberries

Day 14

- Breakfast: Peanut Butter and Banana Overnight Oats
- Lunch: Roasted Beet and Goat Cheese Salad
- Dinner: Chickpea Curry with Brown Rice
- Snack: Fruit Kabobs
- Dessert: Sweet Potato Brownies

Week 3:

Day 15

- Breakfast: Lentil Breakfast Patties
- Lunch: Veggie Quesadillas with Salsa
- Dinner: Vegetable Paella
- Snack: Kale Chips
- Dessert: Raspberry Chia Jam Bars

Day 16

- Breakfast: Veggie Scramble with Tofu
- Lunch: Chickpea and Avocado Salad
- Dinner: Eggplant Parmesan
- Snack: Roasted Chickpeas
- Dessert: Apple Cinnamon Oat Bars

Day 17

- Breakfast: Berry Oatmeal with Chia Seeds
- Lunch: Lentil Soup with Vegetables
- Dinner: Vegetable Stir-Fry with Tofu
- Snack: Veggie Sticks with Hummus
- Dessert: Baked Pears with Cinnamon

Day 18

- Breakfast: Spinach and Mushroom Omelette
- Lunch: Quinoa and Black Bean Salad
- Dinner: Spinach and Ricotta Stuffed Shells
- Snack: Baked Zucchini Chips
- Dessert: Greek Yogurt with Honey and Berries

Day 19

- Breakfast: Whole Grain Pancakes with Almond Butter
- Lunch: Grilled Veggie Wraps
- Dinner: Black Bean and Sweet Potato Enchiladas
- Snack: Edamame with Sea Salt
- Dessert: Vegan Chocolate Avocado Mousse

Day 20

- Breakfast: Greek Yogurt Parfait with Mixed Berries
- Lunch: Spinach and Feta Stuffed Peppers

- Dinner: Veggie Burger with Whole Wheat Bun
- Snack: Apple Slices with Almond Butter
- Dessert: Chia Seed Pudding with Mango

Day 21

- Breakfast: Avocado Toast with Tomato and Basil
- Lunch: Tomato and Basil Soup
- Dinner: Stuffed Bell Peppers with Quinoa
- Snack: Cucumber and Tomato Salad
- Dessert: Mixed Berry Sorbet

Week 4:

Day 22

- Breakfast: Quinoa Breakfast Bowl with Apples and Cinnamon
- Lunch: Veggie Sushi Rolls
- Dinner: Cauliflower Pizza with Veggie Toppings
- Snack: Spinach Artichoke Dip with Whole Grain Crackers
- Dessert: Almond Flour Cookies

Day 23

- Breakfast: Smoothie Bowl with Nuts and Seeds
- Lunch: Greek Salad with Tofu

- Dinner: Ratatouille with Brown Rice
- Snack: Veggie Spring Rolls
- Dessert: Frozen Banana Pops

Day 24

- Breakfast: Sweet Potato Hash with Bell Peppers
- Lunch: Hummus and Veggie Sandwich
- Dinner: Lentil Tacos with Avocado Salsa
- Snack: Sweet Potato Fries
- Dessert: Coconut Macaroons

Day 25

- Breakfast: Cottage Cheese and Fruit Salad
- Lunch: Zucchini Noodles with Pesto
- Dinner: Baked Ziti with Spinach
- Snack: Guacamole with Veggie Dippers
- Dessert: Pumpkin Spice Energy Balls

Day 26

- Breakfast: Vegan Banana Muffins
- Lunch: Stuffed Acorn Squash
- Dinner: Butternut Squash Risotto
- Snack: Mini Caprese Skewers
- Dessert: Lemon Chia Seed Muffins

Day 27

- Breakfast: Whole Wheat Waffles with Fresh Berries
- Lunch: Mushroom and Barley Stew
- Dinner: Broccoli and Cheddar Stuffed Potatoes
- Snack: Carrot and Oat Cookies
- Dessert: Fruit Salad with Mint

Day 28

- Breakfast: Chia Seed Pudding with Coconut Milk
- Lunch: Caprese Salad with Balsamic Glaze
- Dinner: Portobello Mushroom Fajitas
- Snack: Cauliflower Buffalo Wings
- Dessert: Dark Chocolate Dipped Strawberries

Day 29

- Breakfast: Peanut Butter and Banana Overnight Oats
- Lunch: Roasted Beet and Goat Cheese Salad
- Dinner: Chickpea Curry with Brown Rice
- Snack: Fruit Kabobs
- Dessert: Sweet Potato Brownies

Day 30

- Breakfast: Lentil Breakfast Patties
- Lunch: Veggie Quesadillas with Salsa

- Dinner: Vegetable Paella
- Snack: Kale Chips
- Dessert: Raspberry Chia Jam Bars

Chapter 2: Breakfast Recipes

Breakfast is a crucial meal for children with Type 1 diabetes, providing the energy and nutrients necessary to start their day off right. The following vegetarian recipes are designed to be nutritious, delicious, and kid-friendly, ensuring that each meal is balanced and supports their dietary needs.

Veggie Scramble with Tofu

Ingredients:

- 1 block firm tofu, crumbled
- 1 bell pepper, diced
- 1 small onion, chopped
- 1 cup spinach, chopped
- 1 tablespoon olive oil
- 1 teaspoon turmeric
- Salt and pepper to taste

Instructions:

1. Heat olive oil in a pan over medium heat.
2. Add onions and bell peppers; sauté until soft.
3. Add crumbled tofu and turmeric, stir well.
4. Mix in spinach and cook until wilted.

5. Season with salt and pepper.

Nutrition Information (per serving):

- Calories: 180
- Protein: 12g
- Carbohydrates: 8g
- Fat: 12g
- Fiber: 3g
- Sugar: 2g
- Portion Size: 1 cup

Berry Oatmeal with Chia Seeds

Ingredients:

- 1 cup rolled oats
- 2 cups almond milk
- 1 cup mixed berries
- 1 tablespoon chia seeds
- 1 tablespoon honey (optional)

Instructions:

1. Cook oats with almond milk according to package instructions.
2. Stir in chia seeds and let sit for 5 minutes.

3. Top with mixed berries and honey if desired.

Nutrition Information (per serving):

- Calories: 250
- Protein: 7g
- Carbohydrates: 45g
- Fat: 6g
- Fiber: 8g
- Sugar: 12g
- Portion Size: 1 bowl

Spinach and Mushroom Omelette

Ingredients:

- 2 eggs
- 1/2 cup spinach, chopped
- 1/2 cup mushrooms, sliced
- 1 tablespoon olive oil
- Salt and pepper to taste

Instructions:

1. Beat eggs in a bowl.
2. Heat olive oil in a pan over medium heat.

3. Sauté mushrooms until soft, add spinach and cook until wilted.

4. Pour beaten eggs over veggies and cook until set.

5. Fold omelette and season with salt and pepper.

Nutrition Information (per serving):

- Calories: 200
- Protein: 14g
- Carbohydrates: 4g
- Fat: 15g
- Fiber: 1g
- Sugar: 2g
- Portion Size: 1 omelette

Whole Grain Pancakes with Almond Butter

Ingredients:

- 1 cup whole grain flour
- 1 tablespoon baking powder
- 1 cup almond milk
- 1 tablespoon maple syrup
- 1/4 cup almond butter

Instructions:

1. Mix flour and baking powder in a bowl.

2. Add almond milk and maple syrup, stir until smooth.

3. Cook pancakes on a griddle until bubbles form and edges are set.

4. Top with almond butter before serving.

Nutrition Information (per serving):

- Calories: 250

- Protein: 8g

- Carbohydrates: 32g

- Fat: 10g

- Fiber: 5g

- Sugar: 6g

- Portion Size: 2 pancakes

Greek Yogurt Parfait with Mixed Berries

Ingredients:

- 1 cup Greek yogurt

- 1/2 cup mixed berries

- 1 tablespoon honey

- 1/4 cup granola

Instructions:

1. Layer Greek yogurt in a cup.

2. Add mixed berries on top.

3. Drizzle with honey and sprinkle granola.

Nutrition Information (per serving):

- Calories: 300

- Protein: 15g

- Carbohydrates: 40g

- Fat: 8g

- Fiber: 5g

- Sugar: 25g

- Portion Size: 1 parfait

Avocado Toast with Tomato and Basil

Ingredients:

- 1 avocado, mashed

- 2 slices whole grain bread, toasted

- 1 tomato, sliced

- Fresh basil leaves

- Salt and pepper to taste

Instructions:

1. Spread mashed avocado on toasted bread.

2. Top with tomato slices and basil leaves.

3. Season with salt and pepper.

Nutrition Information (per serving):

- Calories: 350

- Protein: 8g

- Carbohydrates: 38g

- Fat: 20g

- Fiber: 10g

- Sugar: 5g

- Portion Size: 2 slices

Quinoa Breakfast Bowl with Apples and Cinnamon

Ingredients:

- 1 cup cooked quinoa

- 1 apple, chopped

- 1 teaspoon cinnamon

- 1 tablespoon maple syrup

- 1/4 cup almond milk

Instructions:

1. Combine cooked quinoa, apple, cinnamon, and maple syrup in a bowl.

2. Pour almond milk over the mixture and stir.

Nutrition Information (per serving):

- Calories: 250
- Protein: 6g
- Carbohydrates: 50g
- Fat: 4g
- Fiber: 6g
- Sugar: 15g
- Portion Size: 1 bowl

Smoothie Bowl with Nuts and Seeds

Ingredients:

- 1 banana, frozen
- 1/2 cup berries, frozen
- 1/2 cup spinach
- 1/2 cup almond milk
- 1 tablespoon mixed nuts and seeds

Instructions:

1. Blend banana, berries, spinach, and almond milk until smooth.

2. Pour into a bowl and top with nuts and seeds.

Nutrition Information (per serving):

- Calories: 250

- Protein: 5g

- Carbohydrates: 45g

- Fat: 8g

- Fiber: 8g

- Sugar: 25g

- Portion Size: 1 bowl

Sweet Potato Hash with Bell Peppers

Ingredients:

- 1 large sweet potato, diced

- 1 bell pepper, diced

- 1 small onion, chopped

- 1 tablespoon olive oil

- Salt and pepper to taste

Instructions:

1. Heat olive oil in a pan over medium heat.
2. Add sweet potato and cook until slightly tender.
3. Add bell pepper and onion, cook until all veggies are tender.
4. Season with salt and pepper.

Nutrition Information (per serving):

- Calories: 180
- Protein: 2g
- Carbohydrates: 30g
- Fat: 7g
- Fiber: 5g
- Sugar: 8g
- Portion Size: 1 cup

Cottage Cheese and Fruit Salad

Ingredients:

- 1 cup cottage cheese
- 1/2 cup pineapple chunks
- 1/2 cup blueberries
- 1 tablespoon honey (optional)

Instructions:

1. Combine cottage cheese with pineapple and blueberries.

2. Drizzle with honey if desired.

Nutrition Information (per serving):

- Calories: 200

- Protein: 15g

- Carbohydrates: 20g

- Fat: 5g

- Fiber: 2g

- Sugar: 15g

- Portion Size: 1 bowl

Vegan Banana Muffins

Ingredients:

- 2 ripe bananas, mashed

- 1 cup whole wheat flour

- 1/4 cup maple syrup

- 1 teaspoon baking powder

- 1/2 teaspoon baking soda

- 1/4 cup almond milk

- 1 teaspoon vanilla extract

Instructions:

1. Preheat oven to 350°F (175°C).

2. Mix bananas, maple syrup, almond milk, and vanilla extract in a bowl.

3. Add flour, baking powder, and baking soda; stir until combined.

4. Pour batter into muffin tins and bake for 20-25 minutes.

Nutrition Information (per serving):

- Calories: 150

- Protein: 3g

- Carbohydrates: 30g

- Fat: 3g

- Fiber: 4g

- Sugar: 12g

- Portion Size: 1 muffin

Whole Wheat Waffles with Fresh Berries

Ingredients:

- 1 cup whole wheat flour

- 1 tablespoon baking powder

- 1 cup almond milk

- 1 tablespoon honey

- 1 cup fresh berries

Instructions:

1. Mix flour and baking powder in a bowl.
2. Add almond milk and honey, stir until smooth.
3. Cook waffles in a waffle iron.
4. Top with fresh berries before serving.

Nutrition Information (per serving):

- Calories: 200
- Protein: 5g
- Carbohydrates: 38g
- Fat: 5g
- Fiber: 5g
- Sugar: 10g
- Portion Size: 2 waffles

Chia Seed Pudding with Coconut Milk

Ingredients:

- 1/4 cup chia seeds
- 1 cup coconut milk
- 1 tablespoon maple syrup
- 1/2 teaspoon vanilla extract

Instructions:

1. Combine chia seeds, coconut milk, maple syrup, and vanilla extract in a bowl.
2. Stir well and refrigerate overnight.
3. Serve chilled.

Nutrition Information (per serving):

- Calories: 200
- Protein: 4g
- Carbohydrates: 20g
- Fat: 12g
- Fiber: 8g
- Sugar: 10g
- Portion Size: 1 cup

Peanut Butter and Banana Overnight Oats

Ingredients:

- 1/2 cup rolled oats
- 1 cup almond milk
- 1 tablespoon peanut butter
- 1 banana, sliced
- 1 teaspoon chia seeds

Instructions:

1. Mix oats, almond milk, peanut butter, and chia seeds in a jar.

2. Add banana slices on top.

3. Refrigerate overnight.

Nutrition Information (per serving):

- Calories: 300

- Protein: 8g

- Carbohydrates: 50g

- Fat: 10g

- Fiber: 8g

- Sugar: 12g

- Portion Size: 1 jar

Lentil Breakfast Patties

Ingredients:

- 1 cup cooked lentils

- 1/2 cup breadcrumbs

- 1 small onion, chopped

- 1 carrot, grated

- 1 tablespoon olive oil

- Salt and pepper to taste

Instructions:

1. Mix lentils, breadcrumbs, onion, and carrot in a bowl.

2. Form mixture into patties.

3. Heat olive oil in a pan over medium heat and cook patties until golden brown.

Nutrition Information (per serving):

- Calories: 180
- Protein: 8g
- Carbohydrates: 25g
- Fat: 6g
- Fiber: 6g
- Sugar: 3g
- Portion Size: 2 patties

Chapter 3: Lunch Recipes

Lunch is an important meal for kids, providing the energy and nutrients they need to stay active and focused throughout the day. For children with Type 1 Diabetes, it's crucial to balance carbohydrates with protein and healthy fats to maintain stable blood sugar levels. The following vegetarian lunch recipes are designed to be nutritious, delicious, and easy to prepare.

Chickpea and Avocado Salad

Ingredients:

- 1 can chickpeas, drained and rinsed
- 1 ripe avocado, diced
- 1 cup cherry tomatoes, halved
- 1/4 red onion, finely chopped
- 2 tablespoons lemon juice
- 1 tablespoon olive oil
- Salt and pepper to taste
- Fresh parsley for garnish

Instructions:

1. In a large bowl, combine chickpeas, avocado, cherry tomatoes, and red onion.

2. Drizzle with lemon juice and olive oil.

3. Season with salt and pepper, and mix gently.

4. Garnish with fresh parsley before serving.

Nutritional Information per serving:

- Calories: 250

- Protein: 8g

- Carbohydrates: 30g

- Fat: 12g

- Fiber: 10g

- Sugar: 3g

- Portion size: 1 cup

Lentil Soup with Vegetables

Ingredients:

- 1 cup green lentils, rinsed

- 1 onion, chopped

- 2 carrots, diced

- 2 celery stalks, diced

- 3 garlic cloves, minced

- 1 can diced tomatoes

- 6 cups vegetable broth

- 1 teaspoon cumin

- 1 teaspoon thyme
- Salt and pepper to taste
- 2 tablespoons olive oil

Instructions:

1. Heat olive oil in a large pot over medium heat. Add onion, carrots, and celery, and sauté until softened.
2. Add garlic and cook for another minute.
3. Stir in lentils, diced tomatoes, vegetable broth, cumin, and thyme.
4. Bring to a boil, then reduce heat and simmer for 30-40 minutes until lentils are tender.
5. Season with salt and pepper to taste before serving.

Nutritional Information per serving:

- Calories: 180
- Protein: 10g
- Carbohydrates: 30g
- Fat: 3g
- Fiber: 12g
- Sugar: 5g
- Portion size: 1 cup

Quinoa and Black Bean Salad

Ingredients:

- 1 cup quinoa, rinsed
- 1 can black beans, drained and rinsed
- 1 cup corn kernels
- 1 red bell pepper, diced
- 1/4 cup chopped cilantro
- 2 tablespoons lime juice
- 1 tablespoon olive oil
- Salt and pepper to taste

Instructions:

1. Cook quinoa according to package instructions and let cool.
2. In a large bowl, combine quinoa, black beans, corn, red bell pepper, and cilantro.
3. Drizzle with lime juice and olive oil.
4. Season with salt and pepper, and toss to combine.

Nutritional Information per serving:

- Calories: 220
- Protein: 8g
- Carbohydrates: 38g
- Fat: 5g
- Fiber: 8g

- Sugar: 2g
- Portion size: 1 cup

Grilled Veggie Wraps

Ingredients:
- 1 zucchini, sliced
- 1 red bell pepper, sliced
- 1 yellow bell pepper, sliced
- 1 red onion, sliced
- 1 tablespoon olive oil
- Salt and pepper to taste
- 4 whole wheat tortillas
- 1/2 cup hummus

Instructions:
1. Toss zucchini, bell peppers, and onion with olive oil, salt, and pepper.
2. Grill vegetables over medium heat until tender.
3. Spread hummus on each tortilla.
4. Add grilled vegetables and roll up the tortillas.

Nutritional Information per serving:
- Calories: 280

- Protein: 7g

- Carbohydrates: 42g

- Fat: 10g

- Fiber: 8g

- Sugar: 5g

- Portion size: 1 wrap

Spinach and Feta Stuffed Peppers

Ingredients:

- 4 bell peppers, tops cut off and seeds removed

- 1 cup cooked quinoa

- 1 cup fresh spinach, chopped

- 1/2 cup crumbled feta cheese

- 1/4 cup chopped red onion

- 1 garlic clove, minced

- 1 tablespoon olive oil

- Salt and pepper to taste

Instructions:

1. Preheat oven to 375°F (190°C).

2. In a bowl, mix quinoa, spinach, feta, red onion, garlic, olive oil, salt, and pepper.

3. Stuff each bell pepper with the mixture.

4. Place peppers in a baking dish and bake for 25-30 minutes.

Nutritional Information per serving:

- Calories: 220

- Protein: 7g

- Carbohydrates: 30g

- Fat: 9g

- Fiber: 5g

- Sugar: 6g

- Portion size: 1 stuffed pepper

Tomato and Basil Soup

Ingredients:

- 6 large tomatoes, chopped

- 1 onion, chopped

- 3 garlic cloves, minced

- 2 cups vegetable broth

- 1/4 cup fresh basil leaves, chopped

- 2 tablespoons olive oil

- Salt and pepper to taste

Instructions:

1. Heat olive oil in a large pot over medium heat. Add onion and garlic, and sauté until softened.
2. Add tomatoes and cook for 10 minutes.
3. Pour in vegetable broth and bring to a boil. Reduce heat and simmer for 15 minutes.
4. Blend the soup until smooth and stir in basil. Season with salt and pepper.

Nutritional Information per serving:

- Calories: 150
- Protein: 3g
- Carbohydrates: 20g
- Fat: 7g
- Fiber: 4g
- Sugar: 12g
- Portion size: 1 cup

Veggie Sushi Rolls

Ingredients:

- 2 cups sushi rice, cooked
- 4 sheets nori (seaweed)
- 1 cucumber, julienned

- 1 carrot, julienned

- 1 avocado, sliced

- 1/2 cup bell pepper, julienned

- Soy sauce for serving

Instructions:

1. Spread sushi rice evenly on each nori sheet.

2. Place cucumber, carrot, avocado, and bell pepper in the center.

3. Roll up the nori tightly and slice into pieces.

4. Serve with soy sauce.

Nutritional Information per serving:

- Calories: 180

- Protein: 4g

- Carbohydrates: 36g

- Fat: 4g

- Fiber: 4g

- Sugar: 2g

- Portion size: 4 pieces

Greek Salad with Tofu

Ingredients:

- 1 block tofu, cubed
- 1 cucumber, diced
- 1 cup cherry tomatoes, halved
- 1/4 red onion, thinly sliced
- 1/4 cup kalamata olives
- 1/4 cup feta cheese, crumbled
- 2 tablespoons olive oil
- 1 tablespoon red wine vinegar
- Salt and pepper to taste
- Oregano to taste

Instructions:

1. In a bowl, combine tofu, cucumber, cherry tomatoes, red onion, olives, and feta cheese.
2. Drizzle with olive oil and red wine vinegar.
3. Season with salt, pepper, and oregano, and toss gently.

Nutritional Information per serving:

- Calories: 250
- Protein: 12g
- Carbohydrates: 10g
- Fat: 20g

- Fiber: 4g

- Sugar: 4g

- Portion size: 1 cup

Hummus and Veggie Sandwich

Ingredients:

- 4 slices whole grain bread

- 1/2 cup hummus

- 1 cucumber, sliced

- 1 tomato, sliced

- 1/2 red bell pepper, sliced

- 1/4 red onion, sliced

- 1 handful spinach leaves

Instructions:

1. Spread hummus on each slice of bread.

2. Layer cucumber, tomato, bell pepper, red onion, and spinach on two slices.

3. Top with the remaining bread slices.

Nutritional Information per serving:

- Calories: 300

- Protein: 10g

- Carbohydrates: 45g

- Fat: 10g

- Fiber: 8g

- Sugar: 6g

- Portion size: 1 sandwich

Zucchini Noodles with Pesto

Ingredients:

- 2 large zucchinis, spiralized

- 1/4 cup basil pesto

- Cherry tomatoes, halved

- Parmesan cheese, grated (optional)

Instructions:

1. Spiralize the zucchinis to create "noodles."

2. Toss the zucchini noodles with basil pesto until evenly coated.

3. Top with cherry tomatoes and grated Parmesan cheese if desired.

4. Serve chilled or at room temperature.

Nutrition Information (per serving):

- Calories: 180

- Protein: 5g

- Carbohydrates: 10g

- Fat: 14g

- Fiber: 3g

- Sugar: 5g

- Portion Size: 1 cup

Stuffed Acorn Squash

Ingredients:

- 2 acorn squashes, halved and seeded

- 1 cup cooked quinoa

- 1 cup black beans, drained and rinsed

- 1/2 cup diced bell peppers

- 1/4 cup chopped cilantro

- 1 teaspoon cumin

- Salt and pepper to taste

Instructions:

1. Preheat oven to 375°F (190°C).

2. Place the halved acorn squashes on a baking sheet, cut side up.

3. In a bowl, mix together cooked quinoa, black beans, bell peppers, cilantro, cumin, salt, and pepper.

4. Spoon the quinoa mixture into the center of each acorn squash half.

5. Bake for 25-30 minutes, or until squash is tender.

6. Serve hot.

Nutrition Information (per serving):

- Calories: 320
- Protein: 10g
- Carbohydrates: 60g
- Fat: 3g
- Fiber: 12g
- Sugar: 3g
- Portion Size: 1 stuffed squash half

Mushroom and Barley Stew

Ingredients:

- 1 tablespoon olive oil
- 1 onion, diced
- 2 cloves garlic, minced
- 8 ounces mushrooms, sliced
- 1 cup pearl barley
- 4 cups vegetable broth
- 1 teaspoon thyme

- Salt and pepper to taste

Instructions:

1. In a large pot, heat olive oil over medium heat. Add diced onion and minced garlic, sauté until softened.
2. Add sliced mushrooms to the pot and cook until they release their juices.
3. Stir in pearl barley, vegetable broth, thyme, salt, and pepper.
4. Bring to a boil, then reduce heat and simmer for 30-40 minutes, or until barley is tender.
5. Serve hot.

Nutrition Information (per serving):

- Calories: 280
- Protein: 8g
- Carbohydrates: 50g
- Fat: 5g
- Fiber: 10g
- Sugar: 3g
- Portion Size: 1 cup

Caprese Salad with Balsamic Glaze

Ingredients:

- 2 large tomatoes, sliced
- 8 ounces fresh mozzarella cheese, sliced
- Fresh basil leaves
- Balsamic glaze
- Salt and pepper to taste

Instructions:

1. Arrange tomato and mozzarella slices on a plate, alternating with basil leaves.
2. Drizzle with balsamic glaze.
3. Season with salt and pepper to taste.
4. Serve chilled.

Nutrition Information (per serving):

- Calories: 250
- Protein: 15g
- Carbohydrates: 7g
- Fat: 18g
- Fiber: 2g
- Sugar: 5g
- Portion Size: 1/2 plate

Roasted Beet and Goat Cheese Salad

Ingredients:

- 4 medium beets, peeled and cubed
- 2 tablespoons olive oil
- Salt and pepper to taste
- 4 cups mixed greens
- 1/4 cup crumbled goat cheese
- Balsamic vinaigrette dressing

Instructions:

1. Preheat oven to 400°F (200°C).
2. Toss cubed beets with olive oil, salt, and pepper.
3. Spread beets in a single layer on a baking sheet and roast for 25-30 minutes, or until tender.
4. Let the beets cool slightly.
5. Arrange mixed greens on a plate, top with roasted beets and crumbled goat cheese.
6. Drizzle with balsamic vinaigrette dressing.
7. Serve immediately.

Nutrition Information (per serving):

- Calories: 220
- Protein: 7g
- Carbohydrates: 20g

- Fat: 14g

- Fiber: 5g

- Sugar: 10g

- Portion Size: 2 cups

Veggie Quesadillas with Salsa

Ingredients:

- 4 whole wheat tortillas

- 1 cup shredded cheese (cheddar or Mexican blend)

- 1 cup mixed bell peppers, diced

- 1 cup black beans, drained and rinsed

- 1/2 cup corn kernels

- 1 teaspoon chili powder

- Salsa for serving

Instructions:

1. Heat a skillet over medium heat.

2. Place one tortilla in the skillet and sprinkle with cheese, bell peppers, black beans, corn, and chili powder.

3. Top with another tortilla.

4. Cook for 2-3 minutes on each side, or until the cheese is melted and the tortillas are golden brown.

5. Repeat with the remaining tortillas and filling ingredients.

6. Cut quesadillas into wedges and serve with salsa.

Nutrition Information (per serving):

- Calories: 320
- Protein: 15g
- Carbohydrates: 45g
- Fat: 10g
- Fiber: 8g
- Sugar: 5g
- Portion Size: 1 quesadilla

Chapter 4: Dinner Recipes

In this chapter, we will explore a variety of delicious, nutritious dinner recipes that are not only satisfying but also packed with essential nutrients. Each dish is thoughtfully crafted to provide a balanced meal, perfect for ending your day on a healthy note.

Eggplant Parmesan

Ingredients:

- 2 large eggplants, sliced into rounds
- 1 cup breadcrumbs
- 1/2 cup grated Parmesan cheese
- 1 cup marinara sauce
- 1 cup shredded mozzarella cheese
- 1/4 cup fresh basil leaves
- 2 eggs, beaten
- Salt and pepper to taste

Instructions:

1. Preheat oven to 375°F (190°C). Line a baking sheet with parchment paper.
2. Dip eggplant slices in beaten eggs, then coat with a mixture of breadcrumbs and Parmesan cheese.

3. Arrange on the baking sheet and bake for 20 minutes, flipping halfway through.
4. Spread a thin layer of marinara sauce in a baking dish, layer with eggplant slices, marinara sauce, and mozzarella cheese.
5. Repeat layers, finishing with mozzarella cheese on top.
6. Bake for 25 minutes until bubbly and golden.
7. Garnish with fresh basil leaves before serving.

Nutrition Information:

- Calories: 320
- Protein: 16g
- Carbohydrates: 42g
- Fat: 12g
- Fiber: 7g
- Sugar: 10g
- Portion size: 1 serving

Vegetable Stir-Fry with Tofu

Ingredients:

- 1 block firm tofu, cubed
- 2 tbsp soy sauce
- 1 tbsp sesame oil
- 1 red bell pepper, sliced

- 1 yellow bell pepper, sliced
- 1 broccoli head, cut into florets
- 2 carrots, julienned
- 2 cloves garlic, minced
- 1 tbsp grated ginger
- 2 tbsp hoisin sauce
- 1 tbsp cornstarch mixed with 2 tbsp water

Instructions:

1. Marinate tofu in soy sauce for 10 minutes.
2. Heat sesame oil in a large skillet over medium-high heat. Add tofu and cook until golden brown. Remove and set aside.
3. In the same skillet, add garlic and ginger, sauté for 1 minute.
4. Add bell peppers, broccoli, and carrots, stir-fry for 5-7 minutes.
5. Return tofu to the skillet, add hoisin sauce and cornstarch mixture, stir until thickened.
6. Serve hot over steamed rice or noodles.

Nutrition Information:

- Calories: 280
- Protein: 15g
- Carbohydrates: 30g

- Fat: 12g

- Fiber: 8g

- Sugar: 8g

- Portion size: 1 serving

Spinach and Ricotta Stuffed Shells

Ingredients:

- 20 jumbo pasta shells

- 2 cups ricotta cheese

- 1 cup cooked spinach, chopped

- 1/2 cup grated Parmesan cheese

- 1 egg, beaten

- 2 cups marinara sauce

- 1 cup shredded mozzarella cheese

- Salt and pepper to taste

Instructions:

1. Preheat oven to 375°F (190°C). Cook pasta shells according to package instructions, drain.

2. In a bowl, mix ricotta, spinach, Parmesan cheese, egg, salt, and pepper.

3. Fill each pasta shell with the ricotta mixture.

4. Spread 1 cup marinara sauce in a baking dish, arrange stuffed shells on top.

5. Pour remaining marinara sauce over shells, sprinkle with mozzarella cheese.

6. Cover with foil and bake for 25 minutes. Remove foil and bake for an additional 10 minutes.

7. Serve hot, garnished with fresh basil if desired.

Nutrition Information:

- Calories: 360
- Protein: 22g
- Carbohydrates: 40g
- Fat: 14g
- Fiber: 5g
- Sugar: 8g
- Portion size: 1 serving

Black Bean and Sweet Potato Enchiladas

Ingredients:

- 2 large sweet potatoes, peeled and diced
- 1 can black beans, drained and rinsed
- 1/2 cup corn kernels
- 1 tsp cumin

- 1 tsp chili powder
- 8 whole wheat tortillas
- 2 cups enchilada sauce
- 1 cup shredded cheddar cheese
- Fresh cilantro for garnish

Instructions:

1. Preheat oven to 375°F (190°C). Cook sweet potatoes in boiling water until tender, drain.
2. In a bowl, mix sweet potatoes, black beans, corn, cumin, and chili powder.
3. Spoon mixture into tortillas, roll up, and place seam-side down in a baking dish.
4. Pour enchilada sauce over tortillas and sprinkle with cheddar cheese.
5. Cover with foil and bake for 20 minutes. Remove foil and bake for an additional 10 minutes.
6. Garnish with fresh cilantro before serving.

Nutrition Information:

- Calories: 420
- Protein: 18g
- Carbohydrates: 65g
- Fat: 12g

- Fiber: 12g

- Sugar: 10g

- Portion size: 1 serving

Veggie Burger with Whole Wheat Bun

Ingredients:

- 1 can black beans, drained and mashed

- 1/2 cup breadcrumbs

- 1/4 cup finely chopped onion

- 1/4 cup grated carrot

- 1 tsp garlic powder

- 1 tsp smoked paprika

- 1 egg, beaten

- 4 whole wheat buns

- Lettuce, tomato, and avocado for topping

Instructions:

1. Preheat grill or skillet over medium heat.

2. In a bowl, combine mashed black beans, breadcrumbs, onion, carrot, garlic powder, smoked paprika, and egg. Mix well.

3. Form mixture into 4 patties.

4. Cook patties on grill or skillet for 5-7 minutes per side until firm and heated through.

5. Serve patties on whole wheat buns with lettuce, tomato, and avocado.

Nutrition Information:

- Calories: 350
- Protein: 15g
- Carbohydrates: 50g
- Fat: 10g
- Fiber: 10g
- Sugar: 6g
- Portion size: 1 serving

Stuffed Bell Peppers with Quinoa

Ingredients:

- 4 bell peppers, tops cut off and seeds removed
- 1 cup quinoa, cooked
- 1 can black beans, drained and rinsed
- 1 cup corn kernels
- 1 cup diced tomatoes
- 1 tsp cumin
- 1 tsp chili powder

- 1/2 cup shredded cheddar cheese
- Fresh cilantro for garnish

Instructions:

1. Preheat oven to 375°F (190°C).
2. In a bowl, mix cooked quinoa, black beans, corn, tomatoes, cumin, and chili powder.
3. Stuff each bell pepper with quinoa mixture.
4. Place stuffed peppers in a baking dish, top with shredded cheddar cheese.
5. Cover with foil and bake for 25 minutes. Remove foil and bake for an additional 10 minutes.
6. Garnish with fresh cilantro before serving.

Nutrition Information:

- Calories: 280
- Protein: 12g
- Carbohydrates: 45g
- Fat: 8g
- Fiber: 10g
- Sugar: 10g
- Portion size: 1 serving

Cauliflower Pizza with Veggie Toppings

Ingredients:

- 1 large cauliflower head, grated
- 1/2 cup grated Parmesan cheese
- 1 egg, beaten
- 1 cup marinara sauce
- 1 cup mixed vegetables (bell peppers, mushrooms, onions)
- 1 cup shredded mozzarella cheese
- Salt and pepper to taste

Instructions:

1. Preheat oven to 400°F (200°C). Line a baking sheet with parchment paper.
2. Microwave grated cauliflower for 8 minutes, let cool, then squeeze out excess moisture.
3. Mix cauliflower with Parmesan cheese, egg, salt, and pepper. Form into a crust on the baking sheet.
4. Bake for 20 minutes until golden and crispy.
5. Spread marinara sauce over crust, top with mixed vegetables and mozzarella cheese.
6. Bake for an additional 10-15 minutes until cheese is melted and bubbly.
7. Slice and serve hot.

Nutrition Information:

- Calories: 250
- Protein: 15g
- Carbohydrates: 20g
- Fat: 12g
- Fiber: 6g
- Sugar: 8g
- Portion size: 1 serving

Ratatouille with Brown Rice

Ingredients:

- 1 eggplant, diced
- 1 zucchini, diced
- 1 yellow squash, diced
- 1 red bell pepper, diced
- 1 yellow bell pepper, diced
- 1 onion, chopped
- 3 cloves garlic, minced
- 2 cups diced tomatoes
- 1 tsp dried thyme
- 1 tsp dried basil
- 1 cup cooked brown rice
- Salt and pepper to taste

Instructions:

1. Heat olive oil in a large skillet over medium heat. Add garlic and onion, sauté until softened.
2. Add eggplant, zucchini, yellow squash, and bell peppers. Cook for 10 minutes, stirring occasionally.
3. Stir in tomatoes, thyme, basil, salt, and pepper. Simmer for 20 minutes.
4. Serve hot over cooked brown rice.

Nutrition Information:

- Calories: 320
- Protein: 8g
- Carbohydrates: 60g
- Fat: 8g
- Fiber: 10g
- Sugar: 14g
- Portion size: 1 serving

Lentil Tacos with Avocado Salsa

Ingredients:

- 1 cup lentils, cooked
- 1 tsp cumin
- 1 tsp chili powder

- 1 tsp garlic powder
- 8 small corn tortillas
- 1 avocado, diced
- 1/2 red onion, finely chopped
- 1/2 cup chopped cilantro
- Juice of 1 lime
- Salt and pepper to taste

Instructions:

1. In a skillet, heat cooked lentils with cumin, chili powder, garlic powder, salt, and pepper.
2. Warm corn tortillas in a dry skillet.
3. In a bowl, combine avocado, red onion, cilantro, lime juice, salt, and pepper to make salsa.
4. Fill tortillas with seasoned lentils and top with avocado salsa.
5. Serve immediately.

Nutrition Information:

- Calories: 280
- Protein: 12g
- Carbohydrates: 45g
- Fat: 8g
- Fiber: 10g
- Sugar: 4g

- Portion size: 1 serving

Baked Ziti with Spinach

Ingredients:

- 12 oz ziti pasta
- 2 cups marinara sauce
- 1 cup ricotta cheese
- 2 cups fresh spinach, chopped
- 1 cup shredded mozzarella cheese
- 1/2 cup grated Parmesan cheese
- 2 cloves garlic, minced
- Salt and pepper to taste

Instructions:

1. Preheat oven to 375°F (190°C). Cook ziti pasta according to package instructions, drain.
2. In a large bowl, mix cooked pasta, marinara sauce, ricotta cheese, spinach, garlic, salt, and pepper.
3. Transfer mixture to a baking dish, top with mozzarella and Parmesan cheese.
4. Bake for 25-30 minutes until bubbly and golden.
5. Serve hot.

Nutrition Information:

- Calories: 400
- Protein: 20g
- Carbohydrates: 60g
- Fat: 12g
- Fiber: 6g
- Sugar: 8g
- Portion size: 1 serving

Butternut Squash Risotto

Ingredients:

- 1 butternut squash, peeled and diced
- 1 1/2 cups arborio rice
- 4 cups vegetable broth
- 1/2 cup white wine
- 1 onion, finely chopped
- 2 cloves garlic, minced
- 1/2 cup grated Parmesan cheese
- 2 tbsp olive oil
- Salt and pepper to taste

Instructions:

1. Heat olive oil in a large pot over medium heat. Add onion and garlic, sauté until softened.
2. Add diced butternut squash and cook for 5 minutes.
3. Stir in arborio rice, cook for 2 minutes until lightly toasted.
4. Add white wine and cook until absorbed.
5. Gradually add vegetable broth, one cup at a time, stirring constantly until absorbed.
6. Continue adding broth until rice is creamy and tender.
7. Stir in Parmesan cheese, salt, and pepper.
8. Serve hot.

Nutrition Information:

- Calories: 350
- Protein: 10g
- Carbohydrates: 60g
- Fat: 8g
- Fiber: 5g
- Sugar: 6g
- Portion size: 1 serving

Broccoli and Cheddar Stuffed Potatoes

Ingredients:

- 4 large russet potatoes
- 1 cup cooked broccoli, chopped
- 1 cup shredded cheddar cheese
- 1/2 cup sour cream
- 2 tbsp butter
- Salt and pepper to taste

Instructions:

1. Preheat oven to 400°F (200°C). Bake potatoes for 1 hour until tender.
2. Cut potatoes in half lengthwise, scoop out the flesh into a bowl, leaving skins intact.
3. Mash potato flesh with butter, sour cream, salt, and pepper.
4. Stir in chopped broccoli and half of the cheddar cheese.
5. Spoon mixture back into potato skins, top with remaining cheddar cheese.
6. Bake for 15 minutes until cheese is melted and bubbly.
7. Serve hot.

Nutrition Information:

- Calories: 300
- Protein: 10g

- Carbohydrates: 50g

- Fat: 10g

- Fiber: 6g

- Sugar: 4g

- Portion size: 1 serving

Portobello Mushroom Fajitas

Ingredients:

- 4 large portobello mushrooms, sliced

- 1 red bell pepper, sliced

- 1 green bell pepper, sliced

- 1 onion, sliced

- 2 tbsp olive oil

- 1 tsp cumin

- 1 tsp chili powder

- 8 small flour tortillas

- 1/2 cup salsa

- 1/2 cup guacamole

- Fresh cilantro for garnish

Instructions:

1. Heat olive oil in a large skillet over medium-high heat. Add mushrooms, bell peppers, and onion. Cook for 10 minutes, stirring occasionally.
2. Add cumin, chili powder, salt, and pepper. Cook for another 5 minutes until vegetables are tender.
3. Warm tortillas in a dry skillet.
4. Serve vegetable mixture in tortillas, topped with salsa, guacamole, and fresh cilantro.

Nutrition Information:

- Calories: 280
- Protein: 8g
- Carbohydrates: 45g
- Fat: 10g
- Fiber: 6g
- Sugar: 6g
- Portion size: 1 serving

Chickpea Curry with Brown Rice

Ingredients:

- 1 can chickpeas, drained and rinsed
- 1 onion, chopped

- 2 cloves garlic, minced
- 1 tbsp curry powder
- 1 tsp ground cumin
- 1 can coconut milk
- 1 cup diced tomatoes
- 2 cups cooked brown rice
- Fresh cilantro for garnish

Instructions:

1. Heat oil in a large pot over medium heat. Add onion and garlic, sauté until softened.
2. Stir in curry powder and cumin, cook for 1 minute.
3. Add chickpeas, coconut milk, and tomatoes. Simmer for 20 minutes until thickened.
4. Serve hot over cooked brown rice, garnished with fresh cilantro.

Nutrition Information:

- Calories: 350
- Protein: 10g
- Carbohydrates: 60g
- Fat: 12g
- Fiber: 8g
- Sugar: 6g

- Portion size: 1 serving

Vegetable Paella

Ingredients:

- 1 cup arborio rice
- 1 red bell pepper, diced
- 1 green bell pepper, diced
- 1 cup green beans, trimmed
- 1 cup artichoke hearts, quartered
- 2 cloves garlic, minced
- 1 tsp smoked paprika
- 1/2 tsp saffron threads
- 4 cups vegetable broth
- 1 lemon, cut into wedges
- Fresh parsley for garnish
- Salt and pepper to taste

Instructions:

1. Heat olive oil in a large skillet over medium heat. Add garlic and cook until fragrant.
2. Add bell peppers, green beans, and artichoke hearts. Cook for 5 minutes.

3. Stir in arborio rice, smoked paprika, saffron, salt, and pepper. Cook for 2 minutes.

4. Gradually add vegetable broth, stirring occasionally, until rice is tender and liquid is absorbed.

5. Serve hot, garnished with lemon wedges and fresh parsley.

Nutrition Information:

- Calories: 340
- Protein: 8g
- Carbohydrates: 60g
- Fat: 8g
- Fiber: 8g
- Sugar: 6g
- Portion size: 1 serving

Chapter 5: Snacks and Appetizers

Snacking can be a delightful and nutritious part of our daily routine. These snack and appetizer recipes offer a variety of flavors and textures, perfect for any time of day. From crunchy chickpeas to refreshing fruit kabobs, each recipe is designed to be easy to prepare and healthy.

Roasted Chickpeas

Ingredients:

- 1 can chickpeas, drained and rinsed
- 1 tbsp olive oil
- 1 tsp paprika
- 1/2 tsp garlic powder
- 1/2 tsp salt

Instructions:

1. Preheat oven to 400°F (200°C).
2. Toss chickpeas with olive oil, paprika, garlic powder, and salt.
3. Spread on a baking sheet and roast for 20-25 minutes, shaking the pan halfway through.

Nutrition Information:

- Calories: 120
- Protein: 6g
- Carbohydrates: 20g
- Fat: 3g
- Fiber: 6g
- Sugar: 1g
- Portion Size: 1/2 cup

Veggie Sticks with Hummus

Ingredients:

- 2 carrots, cut into sticks
- 2 celery stalks, cut into sticks
- 1 cucumber, cut into sticks
- 1 cup hummus

Instructions:

1. Arrange the veggie sticks on a platter.
2. Serve with a bowl of hummus for dipping.

Nutrition Information:

- Calories: 150
- Protein: 5g

- Carbohydrates: 15g

- Fat: 8g

- Fiber: 6g

- Sugar: 5g

- Portion Size: 1 cup veggies with 1/4 cup hummus

Baked Zucchini Chips

Ingredients:

- 2 zucchinis, thinly sliced

- 1 tbsp olive oil

- 1/4 tsp salt

- 1/4 tsp pepper

Instructions:

1. Preheat oven to 225°F (110°C).

2. Toss zucchini slices with olive oil, salt, and pepper.

3. Arrange on a baking sheet and bake for 1.5-2 hours until crispy.

Nutrition Information:

- Calories: 90

- Protein: 2g

- Carbohydrates: 8g

- Fat: 4g

- Fiber: 2g

- Sugar: 3g

- Portion Size: 1 cup

Edamame with Sea Salt

Ingredients:

- 2 cups edamame (in pods)

- 1 tsp sea salt

Instructions:

1. Boil edamame in salted water for 5 minutes.
2. Drain and sprinkle with sea salt.

Nutrition Information:

- Calories: 120

- Protein: 11g

- Carbohydrates: 10g

- Fat: 4g

- Fiber: 5g

- Sugar: 2g

- Portion Size: 1 cup

Apple Slices with Almond Butter

Ingredients:

- 1 apple, sliced
- 2 tbsp almond butter

Instructions:

1. Arrange apple slices on a plate.
2. Serve with almond butter for dipping.

Nutrition Information:

- Calories: 200
- Protein: 4g
- Carbohydrates: 26g
- Fat: 10g
- Fiber: 5g
- Sugar: 18g
- Portion Size: 1 apple with 2 tbsp almond butter

Cucumber and Tomato Salad

Ingredients:

- 1 cucumber, diced
- 1 cup cherry tomatoes, halved
- 1 tbsp olive oil

- 1 tbsp lemon juice
- Salt and pepper to taste

Instructions:

1. Mix cucumber and tomatoes in a bowl.
2. Drizzle with olive oil and lemon juice, then season with salt and pepper.

Nutrition Information:

- Calories: 80
- Protein: 2g
- Carbohydrates: 10g
- Fat: 4g
- Fiber: 2g
- Sugar: 6g
- Portion Size: 1 cup

Spinach Artichoke Dip with Whole Grain Crackers

Ingredients:

- 1 cup spinach, chopped
- 1 cup artichoke hearts, chopped
- 1/2 cup Greek yogurt

- 1/4 cup Parmesan cheese, grated
- 1 clove garlic, minced
- Whole grain crackers

Instructions:

1. Mix spinach, artichoke hearts, Greek yogurt, Parmesan cheese, and garlic in a bowl.
2. Serve with whole grain crackers.

Nutrition Information:

- Calories: 150
- Protein: 6g
- Carbohydrates: 15g
- Fat: 7g
- Fiber: 4g
- Sugar: 2g
- Portion Size: 1/4 cup dip with 10 crackers

Veggie Spring Rolls

Ingredients:

- 6 rice paper wrappers
- 1 cup lettuce, shredded
- 1/2 cup carrot, julienned

- 1/2 cup cucumber, julienned
- 1/2 cup bell pepper, julienned
- 1/4 cup mint leaves
- 1/4 cup cilantro leaves

Instructions:

1. Dip each rice paper wrapper in warm water to soften.
2. Fill with lettuce, carrot, cucumber, bell pepper, mint, and cilantro.
3. Roll tightly and serve.

Nutrition Information:

- Calories: 100
- Protein: 2g
- Carbohydrates: 20g
- Fat: 0.5g
- Fiber: 3g
- Sugar: 3g
- Portion Size: 2 rolls

Sweet Potato Fries

Ingredients:

- 2 sweet potatoes, cut into fries

- 1 tbsp olive oil
- 1/2 tsp paprika
- 1/2 tsp garlic powder
- Salt to taste

Instructions:

1. Preheat oven to 425°F (220°C).
2. Toss sweet potato fries with olive oil, paprika, garlic powder, and salt.
3. Spread on a baking sheet and bake for 20-25 minutes, flipping halfway.

Nutrition Information:

- Calories: 180
- Protein: 2g
- Carbohydrates: 36g
- Fat: 4g
- Fiber: 5g
- Sugar: 8g
- Portion Size: 1 cup

Guacamole with Veggie Dippers

Ingredients:

- 2 avocados, mashed
- 1/4 cup red onion, finely chopped
- 1/4 cup tomato, diced
- 1 tbsp lime juice
- Salt to taste
- Veggie dippers (carrot sticks, cucumber slices, bell pepper strips)

Instructions:

1. Mix avocados, red onion, tomato, lime juice, and salt in a bowl.
2. Serve with veggie dippers.

Nutrition Information:

- Calories: 200
- Protein: 3g
- Carbohydrates: 12g
- Fat: 18g
- Fiber: 8g
- Sugar: 3g
- Portion Size: 1/4 cup guacamole with 1 cup veggie dippers

Mini Caprese Skewers

Ingredients:

- 20 cherry tomatoes
- 20 small mozzarella balls
- 20 basil leaves
- 2 tbsp balsamic glaze

Instructions:

1. Thread a cherry tomato, mozzarella ball, and basil leaf onto each skewer.
2. Drizzle with balsamic glaze.

Nutrition Information:

- Calories: 100
- Protein: 5g
- Carbohydrates: 5g
- Fat: 6g
- Fiber: 1g
- Sugar: 3g
- Portion Size: 4 skewers

Carrot and Oat Cookies

Ingredients:

- 1 cup rolled oats
- 1/2 cup carrot, grated
- 1/4 cup almond butter
- 1/4 cup honey
- 1 tsp cinnamon

Instructions:

1. Preheat oven to 350°F (175°C).
2. Mix all ingredients in a bowl.
3. Drop spoonfuls onto a baking sheet and flatten slightly.
4. Bake for 10-12 minutes.

Nutrition Information:

- Calories: 120
- Protein: 3g
- Carbohydrates: 18g
- Fat: 5g
- Fiber: 3g
- Sugar: 8g
- Portion Size: 2 cookies

Cauliflower Buffalo Wings

Ingredients:

- 1 head cauliflower, cut into florets
- 1/2 cup hot sauce
- 2 tbsp olive oil
- 1/2 tsp garlic powder

Instructions:

1. Preheat oven to 450°F (230°C).
2. Toss cauliflower florets with hot sauce, olive oil, and garlic powder.
3. Spread on a baking sheet and bake for 20-25 minutes.

Nutrition Information:

- Calories: 100
- Protein: 2g
- Carbohydrates: 10g
- Fat: 6g
- Fiber: 3g
- Sugar: 2g
- Portion Size: 1 cup

Fruit Kabobs

Ingredients:

- 1 cup strawberries
- 1 cup pineapple chunks
- 1 cup grapes
- 1 cup melon balls

Instructions:

1. Thread fruits onto skewers in any pattern.
2. Serve chilled.

Nutrition Information:

- Calories: 50
- Protein: 1g
- Carbohydrates: 12g
- Fat: 0g
- Fiber: 2g
- Sugar: 10g
- Portion Size: 2 skewers

Kale Chips

Ingredients:

- 1 bunch kale, torn into pieces

- 1 tbsp olive oil
- 1/2 tsp salt

Instructions:

1. Preheat oven to 300°F (150°C).
2. Toss kale with olive oil and salt.
3. Spread on a baking sheet and bake for 20-25 minutes, until crispy.

Nutrition Information:

- Calories: 70
- Protein: 3g
- Carbohydrates: 7g
- Fat: 4g
- Fiber: 2g
- Sugar: 1g
- Portion Size: 1 cup

Chapter 6: Desserts

Desserts are often the highlight of any meal, providing a sweet ending that leaves a lasting impression. Whether you're looking for something light and fruity, rich and chocolatey, or something in between, this collection of dessert recipes offers a delightful array of options.

Apple Cinnamon Oat Bars

Ingredients:

- 2 cups rolled oats
- 1 cup applesauce
- 1/2 cup honey
- 1 tsp cinnamon
- 1/2 tsp baking powder
- 1/4 tsp salt

Instructions:

1. Preheat the oven to 350°F (175°C). Line a baking dish with parchment paper.
2. In a large bowl, mix all the ingredients until well combined.
3. Press the mixture into the prepared baking dish.
4. Bake for 20-25 minutes or until golden brown.

5. Let cool before cutting into bars.

Nutrition Information (per bar):

- Calories: 150
- Protein: 3g
- Carbohydrates: 32g
- Fat: 2g
- Fiber: 3g
- Sugar: 14g
- Portion Size: 1 bar

Baked Pears with Cinnamon

Ingredients:

- 4 ripe pears, halved and cored
- 2 tbsp honey
- 1 tsp ground cinnamon
- 1/4 cup chopped walnuts

Instructions:

1. Preheat the oven to 375°F (190°C). Place pear halves in a baking dish.
2. Drizzle with honey and sprinkle with cinnamon.
3. Top with chopped walnuts.

4. Bake for 20-25 minutes until pears are tender.

Nutrition Information (per serving):

- Calories: 180
- Protein: 2g
- Carbohydrates: 34g
- Fat: 5g
- Fiber: 6g
- Sugar: 22g
- Portion Size: 1 pear half

Greek Yogurt with Honey and Berries

Ingredients:

- 1 cup Greek yogurt
- 1 tbsp honey
- 1/2 cup mixed berries

Instructions:

1. Spoon yogurt into a bowl.
2. Drizzle with honey and top with mixed berries.

Nutrition Information (per serving):

- Calories: 150

- Protein: 10g

- Carbohydrates: 22g

- Fat: 2g

- Fiber: 3g

- Sugar: 18g

- Portion Size: 1 bowl

Vegan Chocolate Avocado Mousse

Ingredients:

- 2 ripe avocados

- 1/4 cup cocoa powder

- 1/4 cup maple syrup

- 1 tsp vanilla extract

Instructions:

1. Blend all ingredients until smooth.

2. Chill in the refrigerator for at least 30 minutes before serving.

Nutrition Information (per serving):

- Calories: 180

- Protein: 2g

- Carbohydrates: 24g

- Fat: 10g
- Fiber: 7g
- Sugar: 15g
- Portion Size: 1/2 cup

Chia Seed Pudding with Mango

Ingredients:

- 1/4 cup chia seeds
- 1 cup almond milk
- 1 tbsp maple syrup
- 1/2 cup diced mango

Instructions:

1. Mix chia seeds, almond milk, and maple syrup in a bowl.
2. Refrigerate overnight.
3. Top with diced mango before serving.

Nutrition Information (per serving):

- Calories: 200
- Protein: 5g
- Carbohydrates: 30g
- Fat: 8g
- Fiber: 10g

- Sugar: 15g
- Portion Size: 1 bowl

Mixed Berry Sorbet

Ingredients:

- 3 cups mixed berries (frozen)
- 1/4 cup honey
- 1 tbsp lemon juice

Instructions:

1. Blend all ingredients until smooth.
2. Freeze for at least 2 hours before serving.

Nutrition Information (per serving):

- Calories: 100
- Protein: 1g
- Carbohydrates: 26g
- Fat: 0g
- Fiber: 4g
- Sugar: 20g
- Portion Size: 1/2 cup

Almond Flour Cookies

Ingredients:

- 2 cups almond flour
- 1/4 cup honey
- 1/4 cup coconut oil, melted
- 1 tsp vanilla extract

Instructions:

1. Preheat the oven to 350°F (175°C). Line a baking sheet with parchment paper.
2. Mix all ingredients in a bowl until dough forms.
3. Roll into balls and flatten slightly on the baking sheet.
4. Bake for 10-12 minutes until golden brown.

Nutrition Information (per cookie):

- Calories: 120
- Protein: 3g
- Carbohydrates: 8g
- Fat: 10g
- Fiber: 2g
- Sugar: 5g
- Portion Size: 1 cookie

Frozen Banana Pops

Ingredients:

- 2 bananas, cut in half
- 1/2 cup dark chocolate chips, melted
- 1/4 cup chopped nuts

Instructions:

1. Insert popsicle sticks into banana halves.
2. Dip bananas into melted chocolate and roll in chopped nuts.
3. Freeze for at least 2 hours before serving.

Nutrition Information (per pop):

- Calories: 150
- Protein: 2g
- Carbohydrates: 24g
- Fat: 6g
- Fiber: 3g
- Sugar: 15g
- Portion Size: 1 pop

Coconut Macaroons

Ingredients:

- 2 cups shredded coconut

- 1/2 cup sweetened condensed milk
- 1 tsp vanilla extract

Instructions:

1. Preheat the oven to 350°F (175°C). Line a baking sheet with parchment paper.
2. Mix all ingredients in a bowl until well combined.
3. Drop spoonfuls onto the baking sheet.
4. Bake for 15-20 minutes until golden brown.

Nutrition Information (per macaroon):

- Calories: 100
- Protein: 1g
- Carbohydrates: 12g
- Fat: 5g
- Fiber: 1g
- Sugar: 10g
- Portion Size: 1 macaroon

Pumpkin Spice Energy Balls

Ingredients:

- 1 cup rolled oats
- 1/2 cup pumpkin puree

- 1/4 cup honey

- 1 tsp pumpkin pie spice

Instructions:

1. Mix all ingredients in a bowl until well combined.
2. Roll into balls and refrigerate for at least 1 hour before serving.

Nutrition Information (per ball):

- Calories: 80
- Protein: 2g
- Carbohydrates: 14g
- Fat: 2g
- Fiber: 2g
- Sugar: 7g
- Portion Size: 1 ball

Lemon Chia Seed Muffins

Ingredients:

- 1 cup whole wheat flour
- 1/2 cup almond flour
- 1/4 cup chia seeds
- 1/2 cup honey

- 1/2 cup Greek yogurt
- 1/4 cup lemon juice
- 1 tsp baking powder

Instructions:

1. Preheat the oven to 350°F (175°C). Line a muffin tin with paper liners.
2. Mix all ingredients in a bowl until well combined.
3. Spoon batter into muffin tin.
4. Bake for 20-25 minutes until a toothpick comes out clean.

Nutrition Information (per muffin):

- Calories: 150
- Protein: 4g
- Carbohydrates: 24g
- Fat: 5g
- Fiber: 4g
- Sugar: 12g
- Portion Size: 1 muffin

Fruit Salad with Mint

Ingredients:

- 2 cups mixed fruit (melon, berries, kiwi, etc.)

- 1 tbsp honey

- 1 tbsp lemon juice

- 2 tbsp fresh mint, chopped

Instructions:

1. Mix all ingredients in a bowl until well combined.

2. Chill in the refrigerator before serving.

Nutrition Information (per serving):

- Calories: 80

- Protein: 1g

- Carbohydrates: 20g

- Fat: 0g

- Fiber: 3g

- Sugar: 16g

- Portion Size: 1 cup

Dark Chocolate Dipped Strawberries

Ingredients:

- 1 cup strawberries

- 1/2 cup dark chocolate chips, melted

Instructions:

1. Dip strawberries into melted chocolate.

2. Place on parchment paper and refrigerate until chocolate hardens.

Nutrition Information (per serving):

- Calories: 120

- Protein: 1g

- Carbohydrates: 20g

- Fat: 6g

- Fiber: 3g

- Sugar: 15g

- Portion Size: 4 strawberries

Sweet Potato Brownies

Ingredients:

- 1 cup sweet potato puree

- 1/2 cup almond butter

- 1/4 cup cocoa powder

- 1/4 cup honey

Instructions:

1. Preheat the oven to 350°F (175°C). Line a baking dish with parchment paper.
2. Mix all ingredients in a bowl until well combined.
3. Pour batter into the prepared dish.
4. Bake for 20-25 minutes until a toothpick comes out clean.

Nutrition Information (per brownie):

- Calories: 140
- Protein: 3g
- Carbohydrates: 20g
- Fat: 6g
- Fiber: 3g
- Sugar: 12g
- Portion Size: 1 brownie

Raspberry Chia Jam Bars

Ingredients:

- 1 cup rolled oats
- 1/2 cup almond flour
- 1/4 cup honey
- 1/2 cup raspberry chia jam (see note)

Instructions:

1. Preheat the oven to 350°F (175°C). Line a baking dish with parchment paper.
2. Mix oats, almond flour, and honey in a bowl until well combined.
3. Press half the mixture into the prepared dish.
4. Spread raspberry chia jam over the base layer.
5. Top with remaining oat mixture.
6. Bake for 20-25 minutes until golden brown.

Nutrition Information (per bar):

- Calories: 160
- Protein: 3g
- Carbohydrates: 22g
- Fat: 7g
- Fiber: 4g
- Sugar: 10g
- Portion Size: 1 bar

Chapter 7: Smoothies

Smoothies are a versatile and delicious way to boost your nutrition and energy levels. They can serve as a quick breakfast, a post-workout replenishment, or a refreshing snack. This chapter offers unique smoothie recipes, each packed with different flavors and nutrients.

Green Smoothie with Spinach and Pineapple

Ingredients:

- 1 cup fresh spinach
- 1 cup pineapple chunks
- 1 banana
- 1 cup unsweetened almond milk
- 1 tablespoon chia seeds

Instructions:

1. Combine all ingredients in a blender.
2. Blend until smooth.
3. Pour into a glass and enjoy.

Nutrition Information (per serving):

- Calories: 200
- Protein: 3g
- Carbohydrates: 40g
- Fat: 4g
- Fiber: 6g
- Sugar: 26g
- Portion Size: 1 serving

Berry Blast Smoothie

Ingredients:

- 1 cup mixed berries (strawberries, blueberries, raspberries)
- 1 banana
- 1 cup Greek yogurt
- 1 tablespoon honey
- 1/2 cup water

Instructions:

1. Place all ingredients in a blender.
2. Blend until smooth.
3. Serve immediately.

Nutrition Information (per serving):

- Calories: 250
- Protein: 8g
- Carbohydrates: 48g
- Fat: 3g
- Fiber: 7g
- Sugar: 35g
- Portion Size: 1 serving

Tropical Mango Smoothie

Ingredients:

- 1 cup mango chunks
- 1/2 cup pineapple chunks
- 1 banana
- 1 cup coconut water
- 1 tablespoon flax seeds

Instructions:

1. Blend all ingredients until smooth.
2. Pour into a glass and drink.

Nutrition Information (per serving):

- Calories: 220

- Protein: 2g

- Carbohydrates: 55g

- Fat: 1g

- Fiber: 6g

- Sugar: 38g

- Portion Size: 1 serving

Banana and Peanut Butter Smoothie

Ingredients:

- 1 banana

- 2 tablespoons peanut butter

- 1 cup milk (or almond milk)

- 1 tablespoon honey

- 1/2 teaspoon vanilla extract

Instructions:

1. Add all ingredients to a blender.

2. Blend until creamy and smooth.

3. Enjoy immediately.

Nutrition Information (per serving):

- Calories: 300

- Protein: 9g

- Carbohydrates: 40g

- Fat: 14g

- Fiber: 4g

- Sugar: 25g

- Portion Size: 1 serving

Kale and Apple Smoothie

Ingredients:

- 1 cup kale leaves

- 1 apple, chopped

- 1 banana

- 1 cup orange juice

- 1 tablespoon chia seeds

Instructions:

1. Blend all ingredients until smooth.

2. Serve immediately.

Nutrition Information (per serving):

- Calories: 210

- Protein: 3g

- Carbohydrates: 50g

- Fat: 2g

- Fiber: 7g

- Sugar: 35g

- Portion Size: 1 serving

Strawberry Banana Smoothie

Ingredients:

- 1 cup strawberries

- 1 banana

- 1 cup milk (or almond milk)

- 1 tablespoon honey

Instructions:

1. Combine all ingredients in a blender.

2. Blend until smooth.

3. Serve immediately.

Nutrition Information (per serving):

- Calories: 220

- Protein: 4g

- Carbohydrates: 45g

- Fat: 3g

- Fiber: 5g

- Sugar: 30g

- Portion Size: 1 serving

Carrot Ginger Smoothie

Ingredients:

- 1 cup carrot juice
- 1 banana
- 1/2 inch fresh ginger, peeled
- 1 tablespoon lemon juice
- 1 tablespoon honey

Instructions:

1. Add all ingredients to a blender.
2. Blend until smooth.
3. Serve chilled.

Nutrition Information (per serving):

- Calories: 180
- Protein: 2g
- Carbohydrates: 45g
- Fat: 0.5g
- Fiber: 4g
- Sugar: 30g
- Portion Size: 1 serving

Blueberry Almond Smoothie

Ingredients:

- 1 cup blueberries
- 1 banana
- 1 cup almond milk
- 1 tablespoon almond butter
- 1 tablespoon honey

Instructions:

1. Blend all ingredients until smooth.
2. Pour into a glass and enjoy.

Nutrition Information (per serving):

- Calories: 240
- Protein: 4g
- Carbohydrates: 40g
- Fat: 8g
- Fiber: 6g
- Sugar: 30g
- Portion Size: 1 serving

Avocado and Lime Smoothie

Ingredients:

- 1/2 avocado
- 1 banana
- 1 cup spinach
- 1 cup coconut water
- Juice of 1 lime

Instructions:

1. Place all ingredients in a blender.
2. Blend until smooth.
3. Serve immediately.

Nutrition Information (per serving):

- Calories: 180
- Protein: 3g
- Carbohydrates: 30g
- Fat: 8g
- Fiber: 7g
- Sugar: 15g
- Portion Size: 1 serving

Chocolate Protein Smoothie

Ingredients:

- 1 banana
- 1 scoop chocolate protein powder
- 1 tablespoon cocoa powder
- 1 cup milk (or almond milk)
- 1 tablespoon peanut butter

Instructions:

1. Blend all ingredients until smooth.
2. Serve immediately.

Nutrition Information (per serving):

- Calories: 300
- Protein: 20g
- Carbohydrates: 35g
- Fat: 10g
- Fiber: 5g
- Sugar: 20g
- Portion Size: 1 serving

Orange Creamsicle Smoothie

Ingredients:

- 1 orange, peeled and segmented
- 1 banana
- 1 cup vanilla yogurt
- 1/2 cup orange juice
- 1 tablespoon honey

Instructions:

1. Combine all ingredients in a blender.
2. Blend until smooth.
3. Serve immediately.

Nutrition Information (per serving):

- Calories: 250
- Protein: 6g
- Carbohydrates: 50g
- Fat: 3g
- Fiber: 4g
- Sugar: 40g
- Portion Size: 1 serving

Raspberry Coconut Smoothie

Ingredients:

- 1 cup raspberries
- 1 banana
- 1 cup coconut milk
- 1 tablespoon honey

Instructions:

1. Place all ingredients in a blender.
2. Blend until smooth.
3. Serve immediately.

Nutrition Information (per serving):

- Calories: 220
- Protein: 3g
- Carbohydrates: 35g
- Fat: 8g
- Fiber: 7g
- Sugar: 25g
- Portion Size: 1 serving

Pomegranate Power Smoothie

Ingredients:

- 1/2 cup pomegranate juice
- 1/2 cup Greek yogurt
- 1 banana
- 1/2 cup blueberries
- 1 tablespoon chia seeds

Instructions:

1. Add all ingredients to a blender.
2. Blend until smooth.
3. Serve immediately.

Nutrition Information (per serving):

- Calories: 200
- Protein: 6g
- Carbohydrates: 40g
- Fat: 3g
- Fiber: 6g
- Sugar: 30g
- Portion Size: 1 serving

Peach and Oat Smoothie

Ingredients:

- 1 cup peaches, sliced
- 1/2 cup rolled oats
- 1 banana
- 1 cup almond milk
- 1 tablespoon honey

Instructions:

1. Combine all ingredients in a blender.
2. Blend until smooth.
3. Serve immediately.

Nutrition Information (per serving):

- Calories: 230
- Protein: 5g
- Carbohydrates: 45g
- Fat: 4g
- Fiber: 6g
- Sugar: 20g
- Portion Size: 1 serving

Green Detox Smoothie

Ingredients:

- 1 cup kale
- 1/2 cucumber, sliced
- 1 apple, chopped
- 1/2 lemon, juiced
- 1 cup water

Instructions:

1. Blend all ingredients until smooth.
2. Serve immediately.

Nutrition Information (per serving):

- Calories: 150
- Protein: 2g
- Carbohydrates: 35g
- Fat: 1g
- Fiber: 6g
- Sugar: 25g
- Portion Size: 1 serving

CONCLUSION

In crafting this cookbook, our aim was not only to provide a plethora of delicious recipes but also to empower parents and caregivers in creating nutritious, balanced meals for their vegetarian children with Type 1 Diabetes. Throughout these pages, we've woven together the threads of health, flavor, and variety to offer a diverse array of dishes suitable for every occasion.

From hearty breakfasts to satisfying dinners, from wholesome snacks to indulgent desserts, each recipe has been thoughtfully curated to meet the specific dietary needs of young individuals managing diabetes while embracing the vibrant flavors of vegetarian cuisine. We've strived to make every meal a celebration of wholesome ingredients, ensuring that no compromise is made on taste or nutrition.

As you embark on this culinary journey, we encourage you to approach each recipe with creativity and flexibility, adapting them to suit your child's preferences and dietary requirements. Remember, the kitchen is a space for experimentation and discovery, where each meal presents an opportunity to nourish both body and spirit.

Beyond the realm of recipes, we hope this cookbook serves as a guiding light, illuminating the path to healthier eating habits and fostering a deeper understanding of the intricate relationship between food and well-being. Our journey doesn't end here; rather, it's a stepping stone towards a lifetime of nutritious eating and joyful cooking experiences.

As you savor each bite and witness the smiles of satisfaction around your table, may you find reassurance in knowing that you're not alone on this journey. Together, we can navigate the challenges of managing Type 1 Diabetes with grace and resilience, one delicious meal at a time.

Thank you for entrusting us with the opportunity to accompany you on this culinary adventure. Here's to nourishment, vitality, and the boundless possibilities that await in the kitchen and beyond. Cheers to health, happiness, and the joy of cooking for our beloved children.

www.ingramcontent.com/pod-product-compliance
Lightning Source LLC
Chambersburg PA
CBHW072248260726
48659CB00004BA/1490